Counting your macronutrients (macros) should be one of the first steps within your long-term sustainable health goals. Counting macros goes beyond the surface of your caloric intake each day. This allows you to find the right combination of macros within your daily diet to achieve the best you possible. Understanding how each of the macros fit within your diet, allows you to have a healthier view on your overall daily food intake each day. While counting your macros will hold you accountable, it also allows for the moderate indulgence.

So, what are Macros? First you start with your daily calorie target intake. This will be the foundation for the daily macros. Macros are made up of Fats, Carbohydrates, and Proteins. Each gram of fat is contributed to 9 calories. Each gram of Carbohydrates and Proteins are contributed to 4 calories. Most diets will divide these three macros into certain percentage ranges to use for the baseline target.

Equating specific macros for your daily calorie intake. For a daily macro target of 25% Fat, 50% Carbs, and 25% Proteins on a 2,000 calorie per day diet the following should be used. 2,000 x 0.25 = 500 calories for both Fats and Proteins & 2,000 x 0.50 = 1,000 calories for Carbohydrates. Establish the daily grams of fat per day at 500 calories 500/9 = 55.556. Establishing the daily grams of protein per day at 500 calories 500/4 = 125. Finally establishing the daily grams of carbohydrates per day 1,000/4 = 250. So, on a 2,000 calorie diet with a 25%F, 50%C, and 25%P split this will allow 55.55 grams of fat, 250 grams of carbs, and 125 grams of protein.

Once a daily calorie and macro target has been created it is important to have these goals in mind each day. Each day is to be treated as a new day, there is no "banking" macros for a later date. Just as there is no banking macros, if you are to go over one day, start the next day just as it is, a new day. Soon enough counting your macros will become a normal part of your meal planning and have a lasting impact on your overall view of your daily food intake. Using this macro journal will assist you in tracking your daily food intake to a better lifestyle.

Personal Overview

Date	
Weight	
Left Arm	
Right Arm	
Chest	
Waist	
Hips	
Left Leg	
Right Leg	

Personal Overview Check-in

Date	
Weight	
Left Arm	
Right Arm	
Chest	
Waist	
Hips	
Left Leg	
Right Leg	

Personal Overview Beginning

Date	
Weight	
Left Arm	
Right Arm	
Chest	
Waist	
Hips	
Left Leg	
Right Leg	

Personal Overview Check-in

Date	
Weight	
Left Arm	
Right Arm	
Chest	
Waist	
Hips	
Left Leg	
Right Leg	

Personal Overview Check-in

Date	
Weight	
Left Arm	
Right Arm	
Chest	
Waist	
Hips	
Left Leg	
Right Leg	

Personal Overview Check-in

Date	
Weight	
Left Arm	
Right Arm	
Chest	
Waist	
Hips	
Left Leg	
Right Leg	

Personal Overview Check-in

Date	
Weight	
Left Arm	
Right Arm	
Chest	
Waist	
Hips	
Left Leg	
Right Leg	

Personal Overview Check-in

Date	
Weight	
Left Arm	
Right Arm	
Chest	
Waist	
Hips	
Left Leg	
Right Leg	

Personal Overview Check-in

Date	
Weight	
Left Arm	
Right Arm	
Chest	
Waist	
Hips	
Left Leg	
Right Leg	

Personal Overview Check-in

Date	
Weight	
Left Arm	
Right Arm	
Chest	
Waist	
Hips	
Left Leg	
Right Leg	

Personal Overview Check-in

Date	
Weight	
Left Arm	
Right Arm	
Chest	
Waist	
Hips	
Left Leg	
Right Leg	

Personal Overview Check-in

Date	
Weight	
Left Arm	
Right Arm	
Chest	
Waist	
Hips	
Left Leg	
Right Leg	

Weekly Review

Day	Fats	Carbs	Proteins	Calories	Notes
1					
2					
3					
4					
5					
6					
7					
Target					
Total					
Over/Under					

Weekly Review

Day	Fats	Carbs	Proteins	Calories	Notes
1					
2					
3					
4					
5					
6					
7					
Target					
Total					
Over/Under					

Weekly Review

Day	Fats	Carbs	Proteins	Calories	Notes
1					
2					
3					
4					
5					
6					
7					
Target					
Total					
Over/Under					

Weekly Review

Day	Fats	Carbs	Proteins	Calories	Notes
1					
2					
3					
4					
5					
6					
7					
Target					
Total					
Over/Under					

Weekly Review

Day	Fats	Carbs	Proteins	Calories	Notes
1					
2					
3					
4					
5					
6					
7					
Target					
Total					
Over/Under					

Weekly Review

Day	Fats	Carbs	Proteins	Calories	Notes
1					
2					
3					
4					
5					
6					
7					
Target					
Total					
Over/Under					

Weekly Review

Day	Fats	Carbs	Proteins	Calories	Notes
1					
2					
3					
4					
5					
6					
7					
Target					
Total					
Over/Under					

Weekly Review

Day	Fats	Carbs	Proteins	Calories	Notes
1					
2					
3					
4					
5					
6					
7					
Target					
Total					
Over/Under					

Weekly Review

Day	Fats	Carbs	Proteins	Calories	Notes
1					
2					
3					
4					
5					
6					
7					
Target					
Total					
Over/Under					

Weekly Review

Day	Fats	Carbs	Proteins	Calories	Notes
1					
2					
3					
4					
5					
6					
7					
Target					
Total					
Over/Under					

Weekly Review

Day	Fats	Carbs	Proteins	Calories	Notes
1					
2					
3					
4					
5					
6					
7					
Target					
Total					
Over/Under					

Weekly Review

Day	Fats	Carbs	Proteins	Calories	Notes
1					
2					
3					
4					
5					
6					
7					
Target					
Total					
Over/Under					

Common Food Reference

Food	Fats	Carbs	Proteins	Calories	Notes

Date:

Food	Fats	Carbs	Proteins	Calories	Notes
Target					
Total					
Over/Under					

Date:

Food	Fats	Carbs	Proteins	Calories	Notes
Target					
Total					
Over/Under					

Date:

Food	Fats	Carbs	Proteins	Calories	Notes
Target					
Total					
Over/Under					

Date:

Food	Fats	Carbs	Proteins	Calories	Notes
Target					
Total					
Over/Under					

Date:

Food	Fats	Carbs	Proteins	Calories	Notes
Target					
Total					
Over/Under					

Date:

Food	Fats	Carbs	Proteins	Calories	Notes
Target					
Total					
Over/Under					

Date:

Food	Fats	Carbs	Proteins	Calories	Notes
Target					
Total					
Over/Under					

Date:

Food	Fats	Carbs	Proteins	Calories	Notes
Target					
Total					
Over/Under					

Date:

Food	Fats	Carbs	Proteins	Calories	Notes
Target					
Total					
Over/Under					

Date:

Food	Fats	Carbs	Proteins	Calories	Notes
Target					
Total					
Over/Under					

Date:

Food	Fats	Carbs	Proteins	Calories	Notes
Target					
Total					
Over/Under					

Date:

Food	Fats	Carbs	Proteins	Calories	Notes
Target					
Total					
Over/Under					

Date:

Food	Fats	Carbs	Proteins	Calories	Notes
Target					
Total					
Over/Under					

Date:

Food	Fats	Carbs	Proteins	Calories	Notes
Target					
Total					
Over/Under					

Date:

Food	Fats	Carbs	Proteins	Calories	Notes
Target					
Total					
Over/Under					

Date:

Food	Fats	Carbs	Proteins	Calories	Notes
Target					
Total					
Over/Under					

Date:

Food	Fats	Carbs	Proteins	Calories	Notes
Target					
Total					
Over/Under					

Date:

Food	Fats	Carbs	Proteins	Calories	Notes
Target					
Total					
Over/Under					

Date:

Food	Fats	Carbs	Proteins	Calories	Notes
Target					
Total					
Over/Under					

Date:

Food	Fats	Carbs	Proteins	Calories	Notes
Target					
Total					
Over/Under					

Date:

Food	Fats	Carbs	Proteins	Calories	Notes
Target					
Total					
Over/Under					

Date:

Food	Fats	Carbs	Proteins	Calories	Notes
Target					
Total					
Over/Under					

Date:

Food	Fats	Carbs	Proteins	Calories	Notes
Target					
Total					
Over/Under					

Date:

Food	Fats	Carbs	Proteins	Calories	Notes
Target					
Total					
Over/Under					

Date:

Food	Fats	Carbs	Proteins	Calories	Notes
Target					
Total					
Over/Under					

Date:

Food	Fats	Carbs	Proteins	Calories	Notes
Target					
Total					
Over/Under					

Date:

Food	Fats	Carbs	Proteins	Calories	Notes
Target					
Total					
Over/Under					

Date:

Food	Fats	Carbs	Proteins	Calories	Notes
Target					
Total					
Over/Under					

Date:

Food	Fats	Carbs	Proteins	Calories	Notes
Target					
Total					
Over/Under					

Date:

Food	Fats	Carbs	Proteins	Calories	Notes
Target					
Total					
Over/Under					

Date:

Food	Fats	Carbs	Proteins	Calories	Notes
Target					
Total					
Over/Under					

Date:

Food	Fats	Carbs	Proteins	Calories	Notes
Target					
Total					
Over/Under					

Date:

Food	Fats	Carbs	Proteins	Calories	Notes
Target					
Total					
Over/Under					

Date:

Food	Fats	Carbs	Proteins	Calories	Notes
Target					
Total					
Over/Under					

Date:

Food	Fats	Carbs	Proteins	Calories	Notes
Target					
Total					
Over/Under					

Date:

Food	Fats	Carbs	Proteins	Calories	Notes
Target					
Total					
Over/Under					

Date:

Food	Fats	Carbs	Proteins	Calories	Notes
Target					
Total					
Over/Under					

Date:

Food	Fats	Carbs	Proteins	Calories	Notes
Target					
Total					
Over/Under					

Date:

Food	Fats	Carbs	Proteins	Calories	Notes
Target					
Total					
Over/Under					

Date:

Food	Fats	Carbs	Proteins	Calories	Notes
Target					
Total					
Over/Under					

Date:

Food	Fats	Carbs	Proteins	Calories	Notes
Target					
Total					
Over/Under					

Date:

Food	Fats	Carbs	Proteins	Calories	Notes
Target					
Total					
Over/Under					

Date:

Food	Fats	Carbs	Proteins	Calories	Notes
Target					
Total					
Over/Under					

Date:

Food	Fats	Carbs	Proteins	Calories	Notes
Target					
Total					
Over/Under					

Date:

Food	Fats	Carbs	Proteins	Calories	Notes
Target					
Total					
Over/Under					

Date:

Food	Fats	Carbs	Proteins	Calories	Notes
Target					
Total					
Over/Under					

Date:

Food	Fats	Carbs	Proteins	Calories	Notes
Target					
Total					
Over/Under					

Date:

Food	Fats	Carbs	Proteins	Calories	Notes
Target					
Total					
Over/Under					

Date:

Food	Fats	Carbs	Proteins	Calories	Notes
Target					
Total					
Over/Under					

Date:

Food	Fats	Carbs	Proteins	Calories	Notes
Target					
Total					
Over/Under					

Date:

Food	Fats	Carbs	Proteins	Calories	Notes
Target					
Total					
Over/Under					

Date:

Food	Fats	Carbs	Proteins	Calories	Notes
Target					
Total					
Over/Under					

Date:

Food	Fats	Carbs	Proteins	Calories	Notes
Target					
Total					
Over/Under					

Date:

Food	Fats	Carbs	Proteins	Calories	Notes
Target					
Total					
Over/Under					

Date:

Food	Fats	Carbs	Proteins	Calories	Notes
Target					
Total					
Over/Under					

Date:

Food	Fats	Carbs	Proteins	Calories	Notes
Target					
Total					
Over/Under					

Date:

Food	Fats	Carbs	Proteins	Calories	Notes
Target					
Total					
Over/Under					

Date:

Food	Fats	Carbs	Proteins	Calories	Notes
Target					
Total					
Over/Under					

Date:

Food	Fats	Carbs	Proteins	Calories	Notes
Target					
Total					
Over/Under					

Date:

Food	Fats	Carbs	Proteins	Calories	Notes
Target					
Total					
Over/Under					

Date:

Food	Fats	Carbs	Proteins	Calories	Notes
Target					
Total					
Over/Under					

Date:

Food	Fats	Carbs	Proteins	Calories	Notes
Target					
Total					
Over/Under					

Date:

Food	Fats	Carbs	Proteins	Calories	Notes
Target					
Total					
Over/Under					

Date:

Food	Fats	Carbs	Proteins	Calories	Notes
Target					
Total					
Over/Under					

Date:

Food	Fats	Carbs	Proteins	Calories	Notes
Target					
Total					
Over/Under					

Date:

Food	Fats	Carbs	Proteins	Calories	Notes
Target					
Total					
Over/Under					

Date:

Food	Fats	Carbs	Proteins	Calories	Notes
Target					
Total					
Over/Under					

Date:

Food	Fats	Carbs	Proteins	Calories	Notes
Target					
Total					
Over/Under					

Date:

Food	Fats	Carbs	Proteins	Calories	Notes
Target					
Total					
Over/Under					

Date:

Food	Fats	Carbs	Proteins	Calories	Notes
Target					
Total					
Over/Under					

Date:

Food	Fats	Carbs	Proteins	Calories	Notes
Target					
Total					
Over/Under					

Date:

Food	Fats	Carbs	Proteins	Calories	Notes
Target					
Total					
Over/Under					

Date:

Food	Fats	Carbs	Proteins	Calories	Notes
Target					
Total					
Over/Under					

Date:

Food	Fats	Carbs	Proteins	Calories	Notes
Target					
Total					
Over/Under					

Date:

Food	Fats	Carbs	Proteins	Calories	Notes
Target					
Total					
Over/Under					

Date:

Food	Fats	Carbs	Proteins	Calories	Notes
Target					
Total					
Over/Under					

Date:

Food	Fats	Carbs	Proteins	Calories	Notes
Target					
Total					
Over/Under					

Date:

Food	Fats	Carbs	Proteins	Calories	Notes
Target					
Total					
Over/Under					

Date:

Food	Fats	Carbs	Proteins	Calories	Notes
Target					
Total					
Over/Under					

Date:

Food	Fats	Carbs	Proteins	Calories	Notes
Target					
Total					
Over/Under